SHRINKS and other LUNATICS

BY HOWARD DANZIGER

GREETING BOOKS™
Bayside, New York

Dedicated to:
Lori, Zachary and Brandon

To: ______________________________

From: ___________________________

GREETING BOOKS™

Published by

Once Upon A Planet, Inc.
Box 220
Bayside, New York 11361

Illustrations by Anthony D. Tarsia
Designed by Alis Jordan

Once Upon A Planet is a registered trademark.
Printed in the United States of America.

First printing: March 1982
J I H G
ISBN 0-88009-020-0

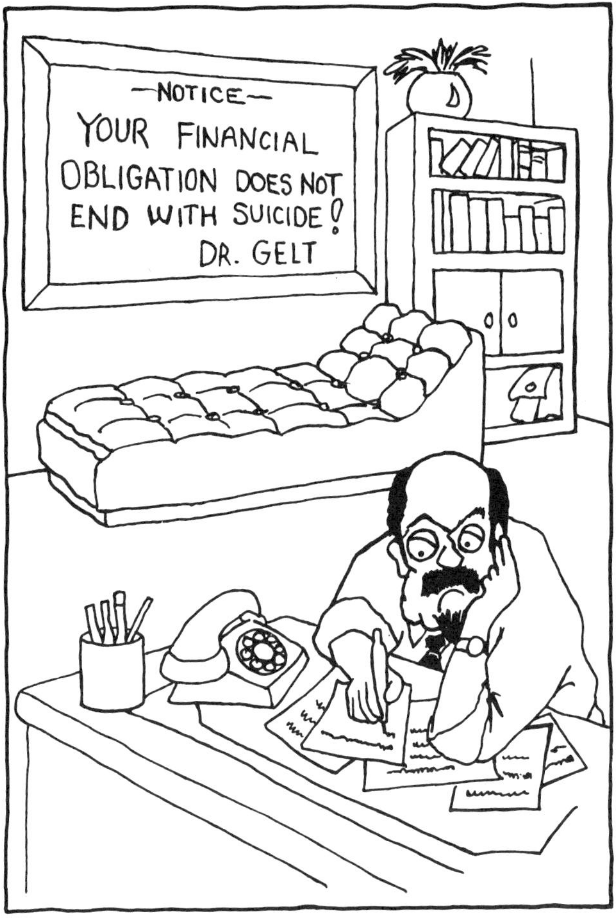
—NOTICE—
YOUR FINANCIAL OBLIGATION DOES NOT END WITH SUICIDE!
DR. GELT

About the Author

Howard Danziger was born in the Bronx on October 20th, 1938. When he was twelve years old, he ran away from the circus to live at home. This upset his parents a lot. They thought he was out of their lives for good. Mom and Dad decided that young Howard needed careful mental supervision...immediately!

Howard was put under the care of the noted Park Avenue psychiatrist, Dr. Segoornisht Helfen. When the young lad asked Dr. Helfen, "How soon will I be cured?" the sympathetic doctor replied, "As soon as you run out of money."

Nowadays, Mr. Danziger spends most of his leisure time trying to figure out the difference between Fernando Lamas and Ricardo Montalban. At this writing, he is currently working on his first novel entitled...*If Lincoln Were Alive Today Would He Take The Bridge Or The Tunnel?*

Mr. Danziger has two goals in life. The first is to win the Nobel Prize for Peace. The second is to be a janitor in the Chrysler Building.

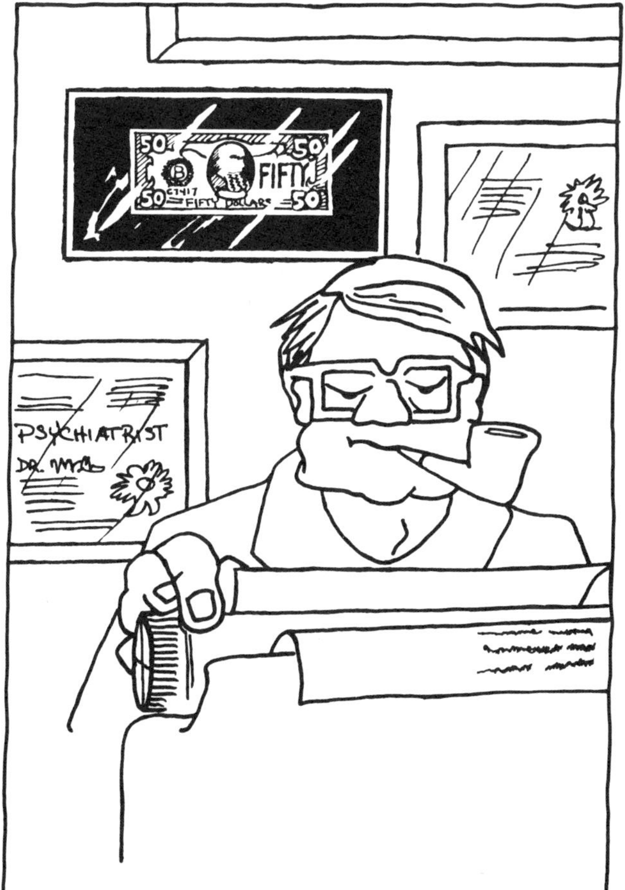

50
50
FIFTY
50
FIFTY DOLLARS
50
PSYCHIATRIST

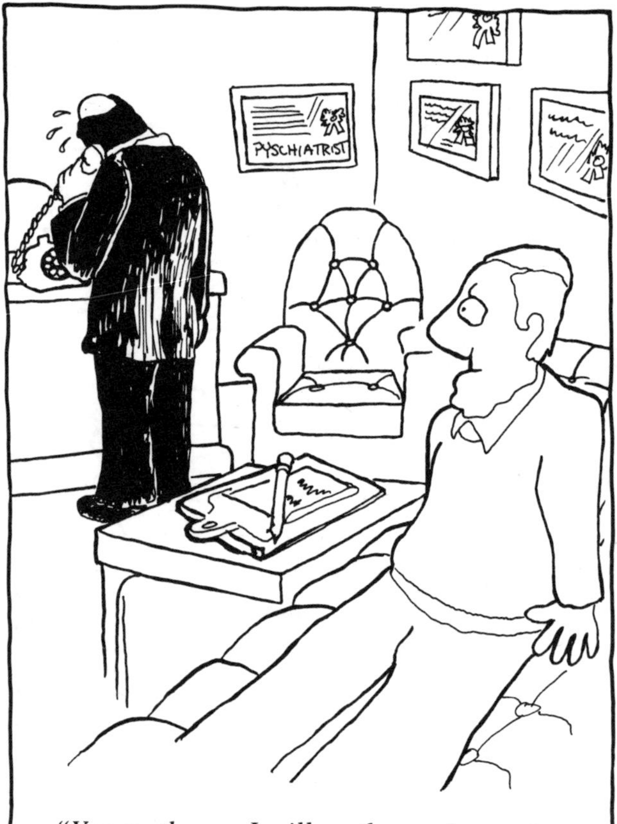

"Yes mother....I will mother....I promise mother....anything you say mother."

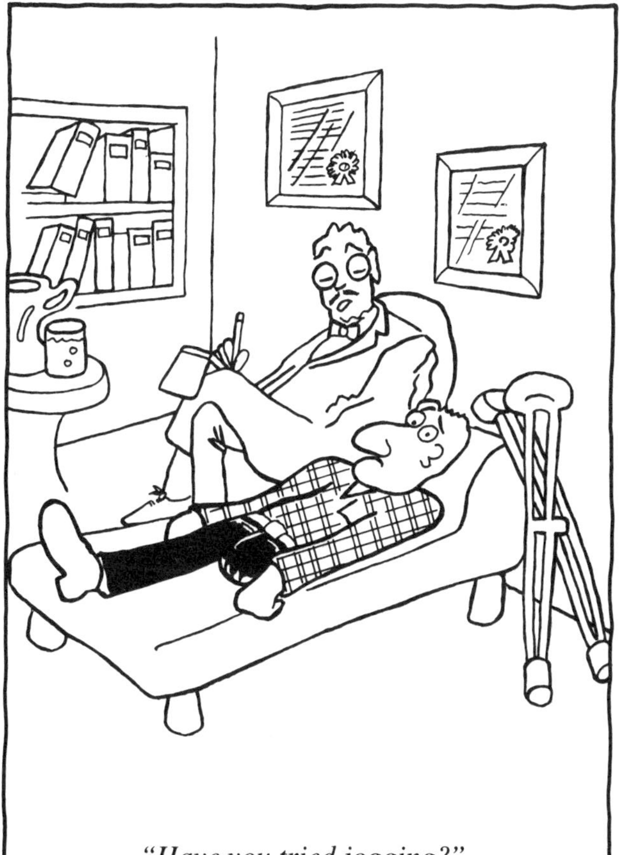

"Have you tried jogging?"

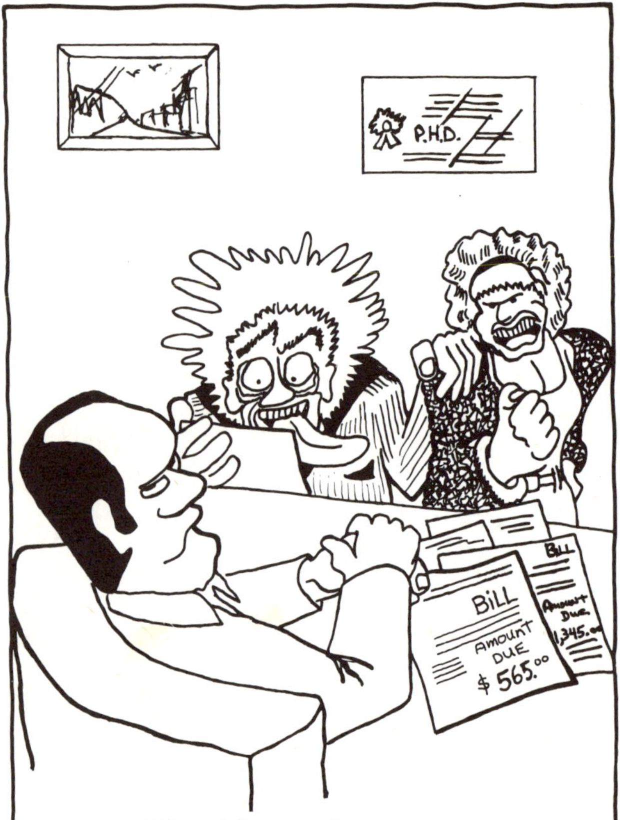

"Now I know what you mean by shock therapy."

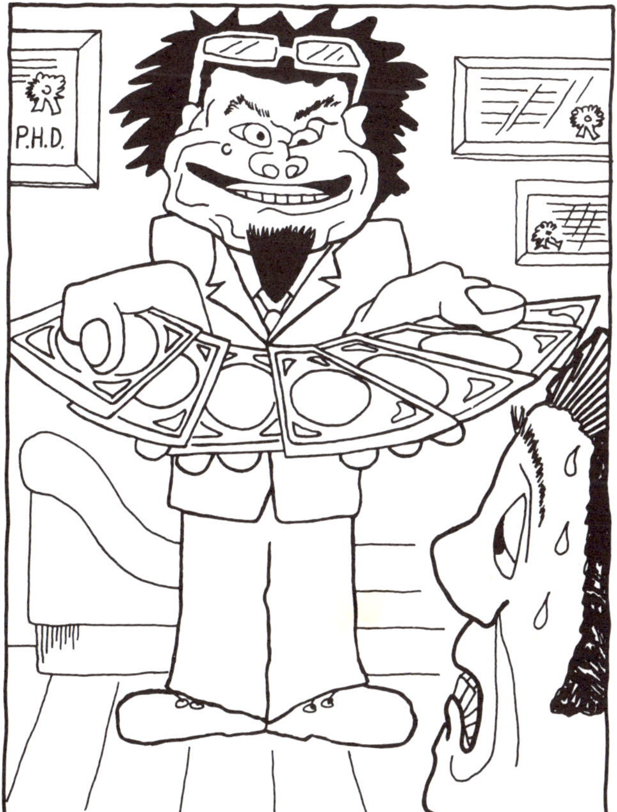

"We'll get to your nervous breakdown in a second……pick a card."

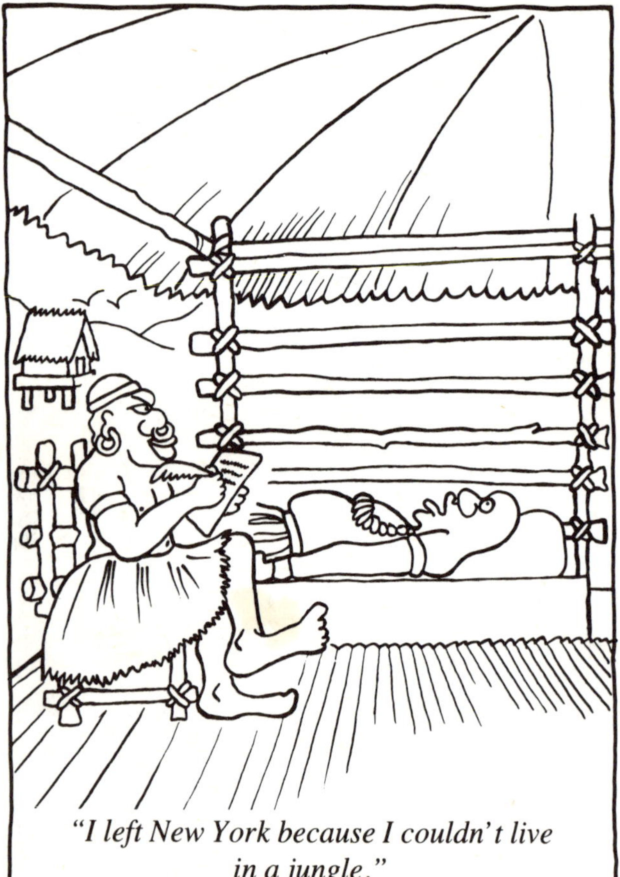

"I left New York because I couldn't live in a jungle."

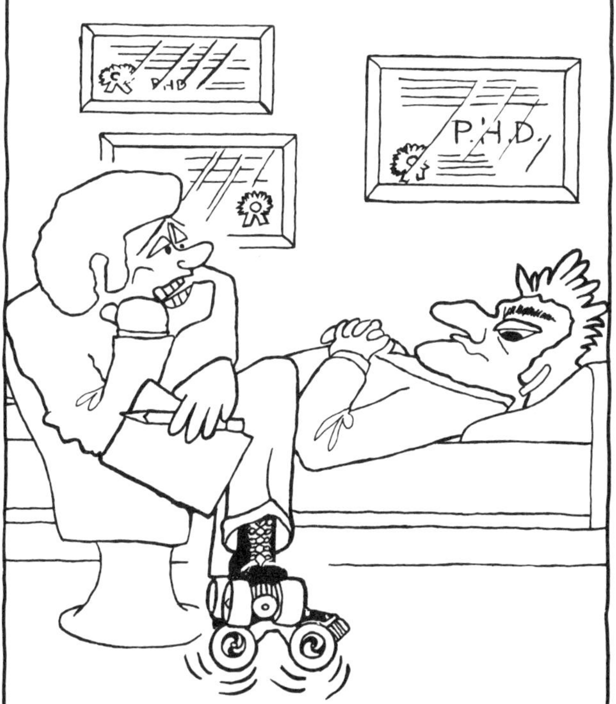

"Nowadays, who's normal?"

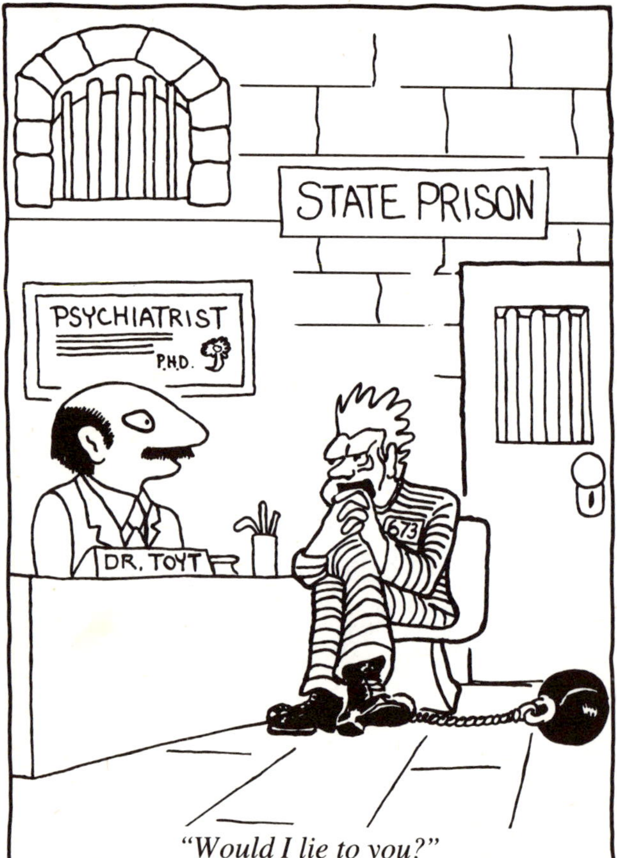

"Would I lie to you?"

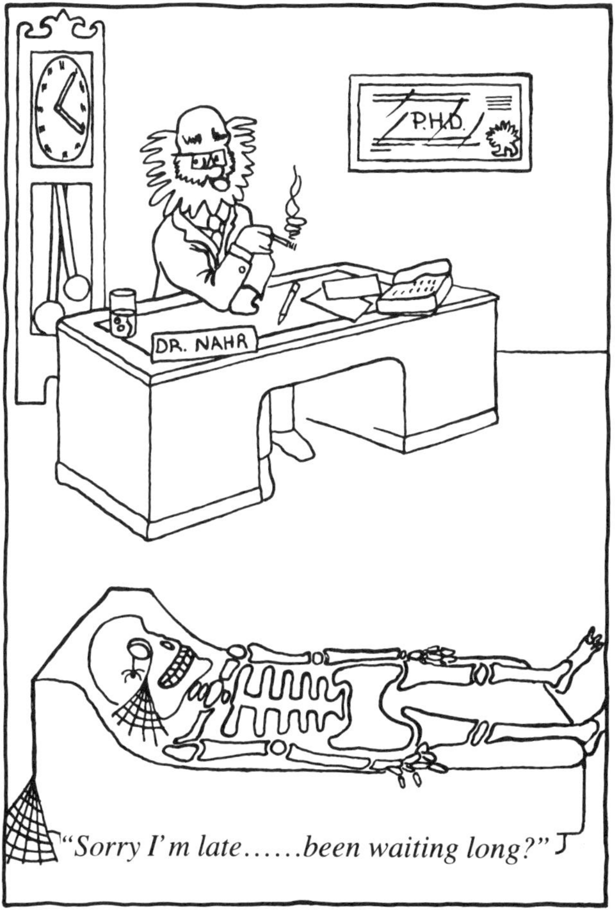

"Sorry I'm late……been waiting long?"

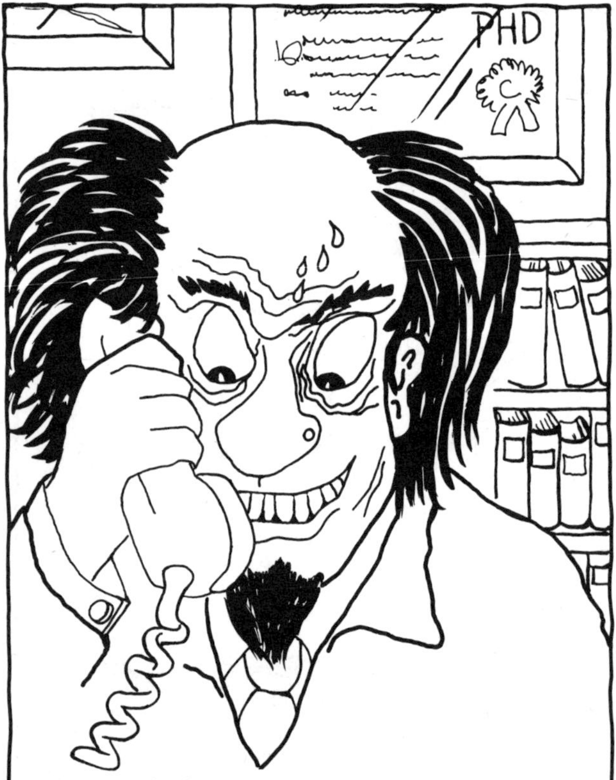

"....and after I penetrate your psyche, the imagery of my phallus will arouse your libido and....hello, hello?"

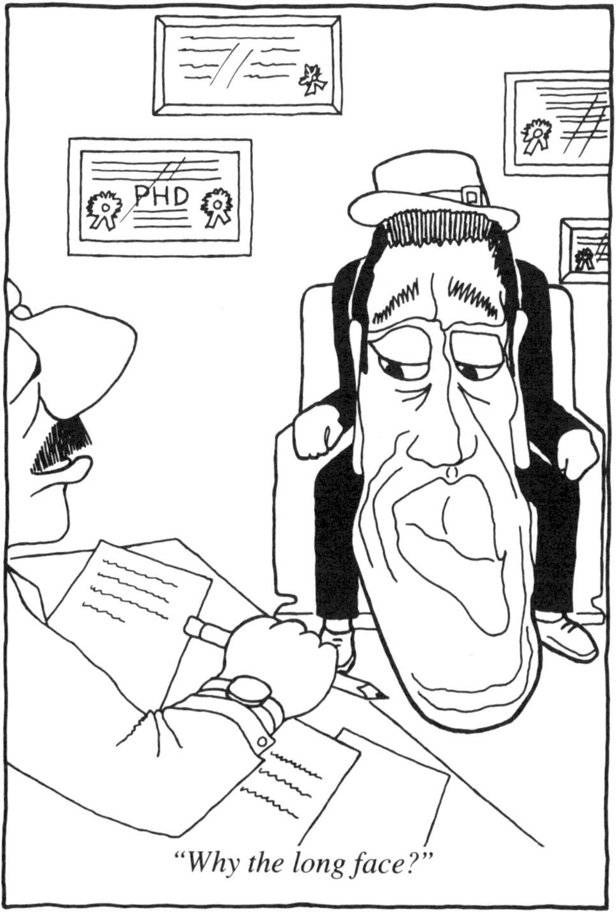

"Why the long face?"

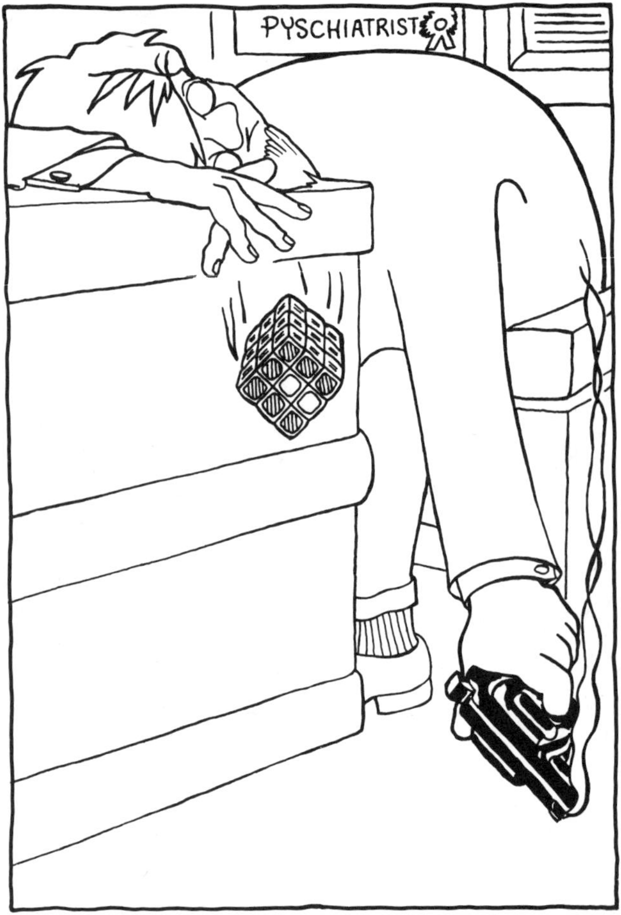
PYSCHIATRIST

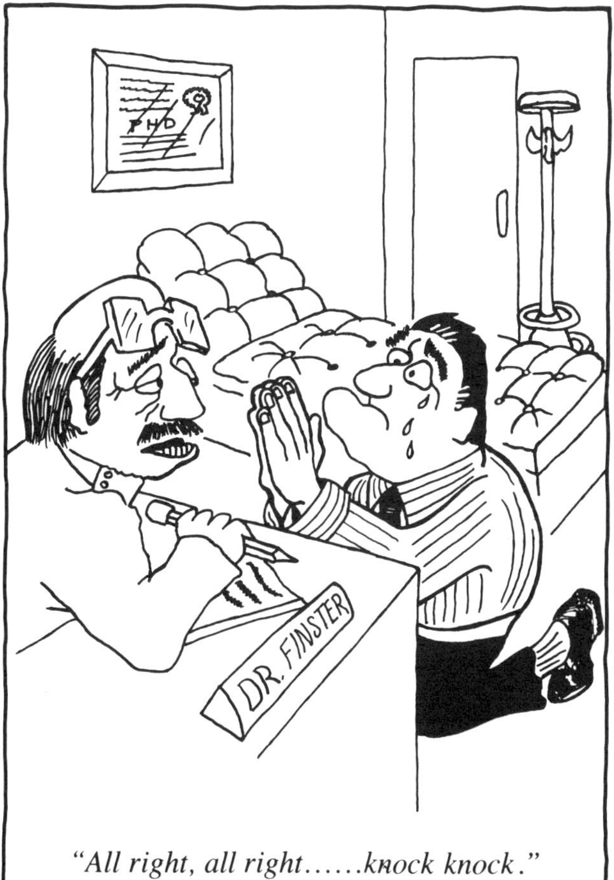

"All right, all right……knock knock."

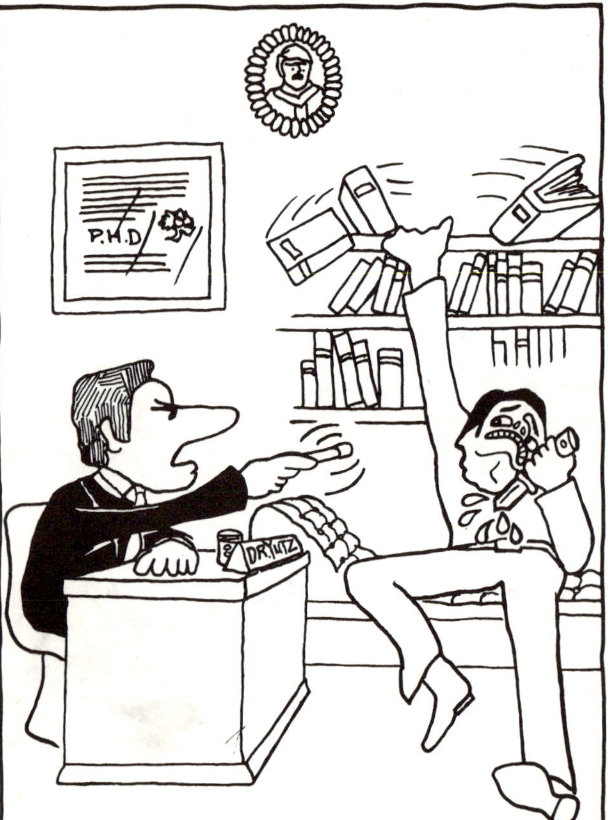

"If you're looking for sympathy, you've come to the wrong place."

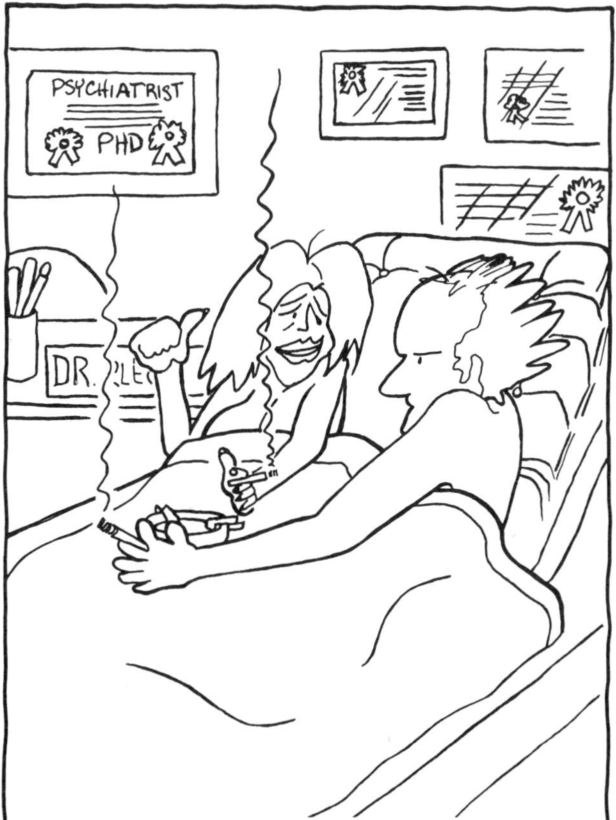

"Wow, ten bucks a session...you're the first shrink that wasn't out to screw me."

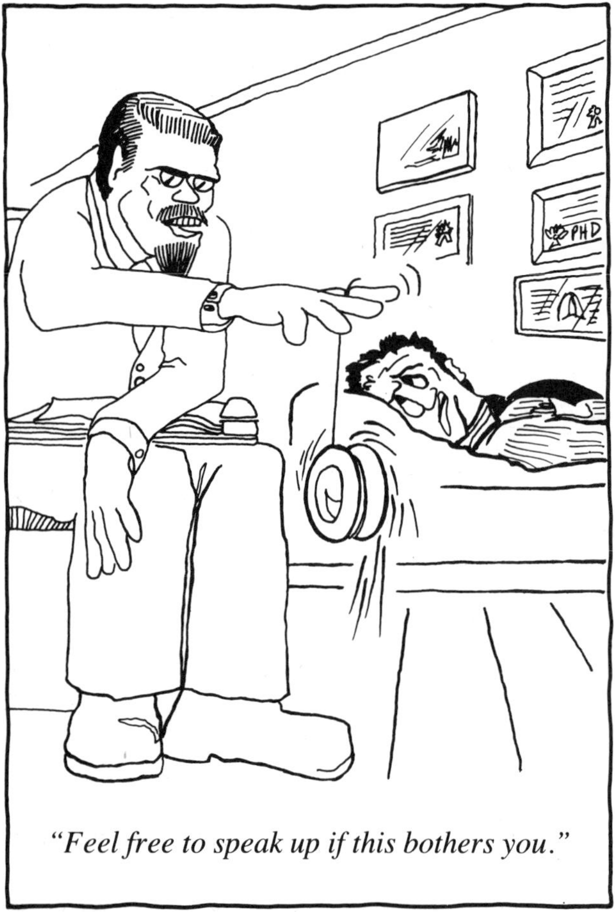

"Feel free to speak up if this bothers you."

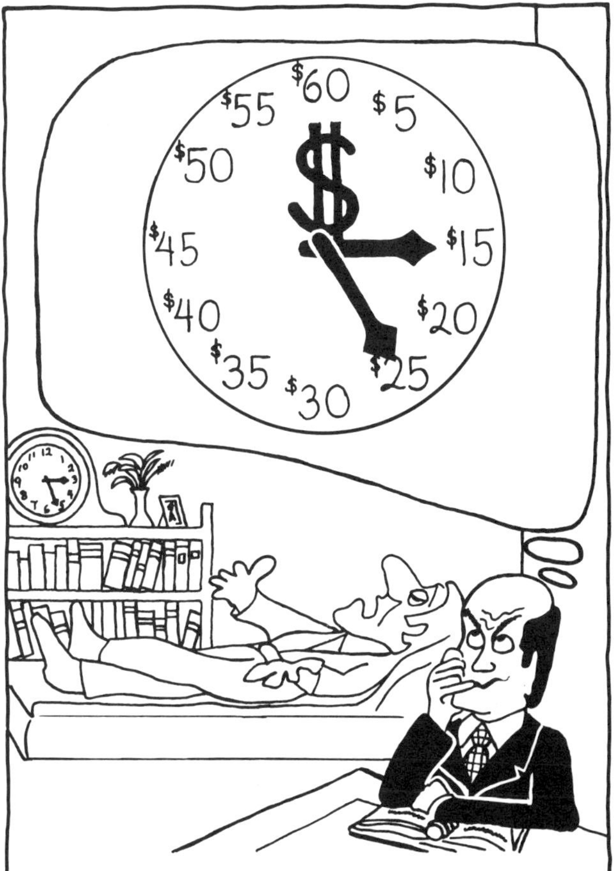
$60
$5
$10
$15
$20
$25
$30
$35
$40
$45
$50
$55

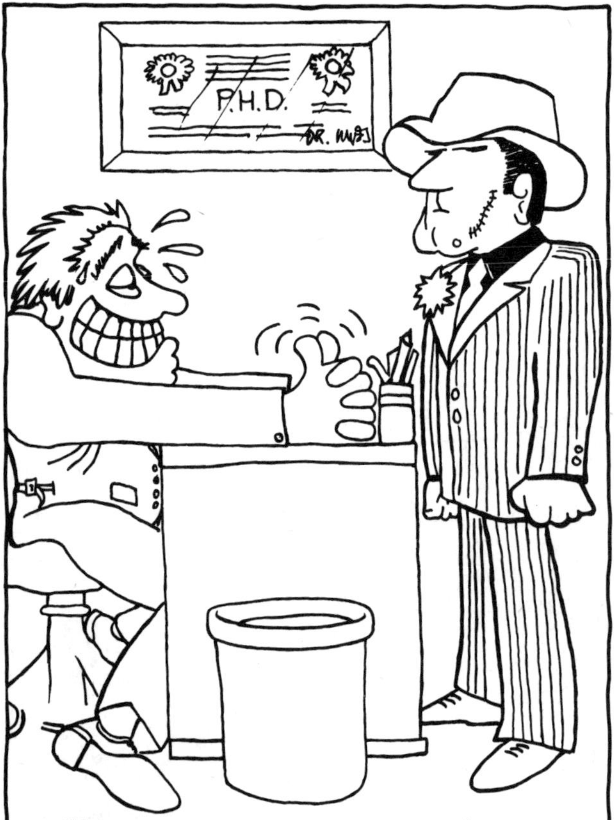

"In your case, you can pay me when you have the money."

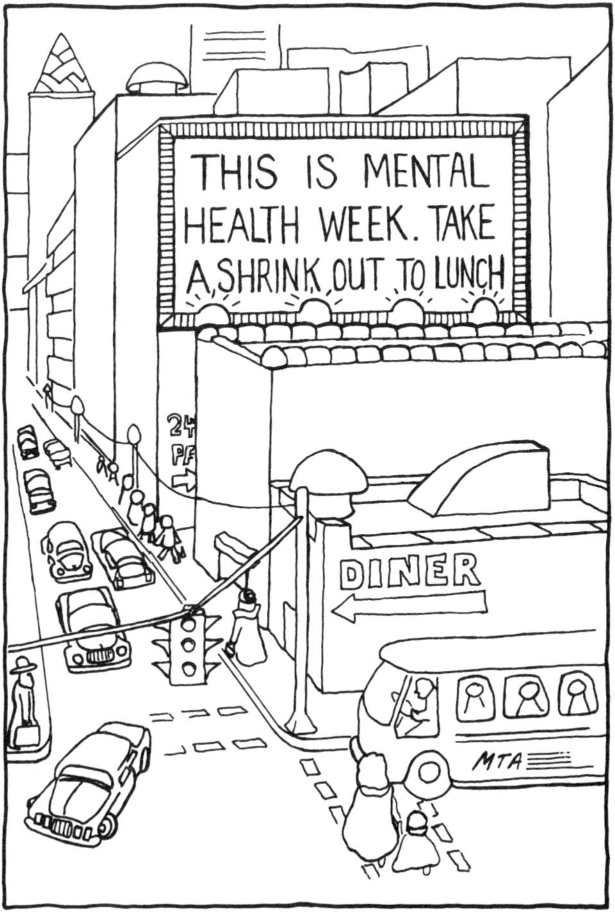
THIS IS MENTAL HEALTH WEEK. TAKE A SHRINK OUT TO LUNCH
DINER
MTA

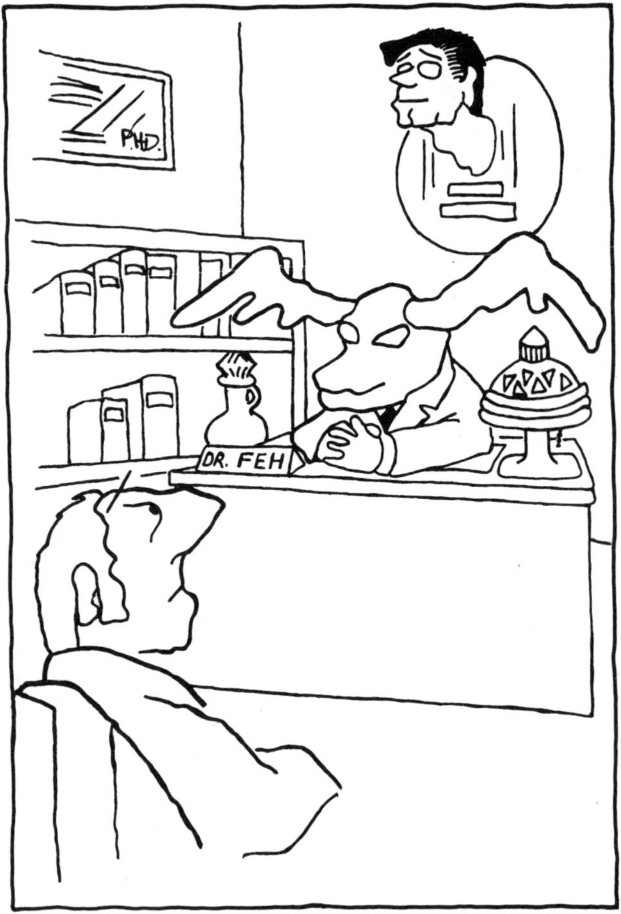
PHD.
DR. FEH

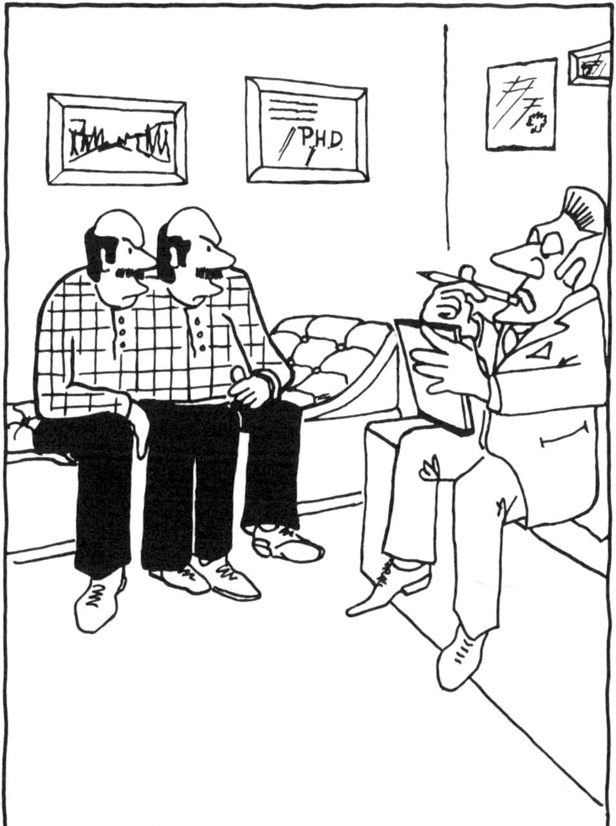

"Have you always been close?"

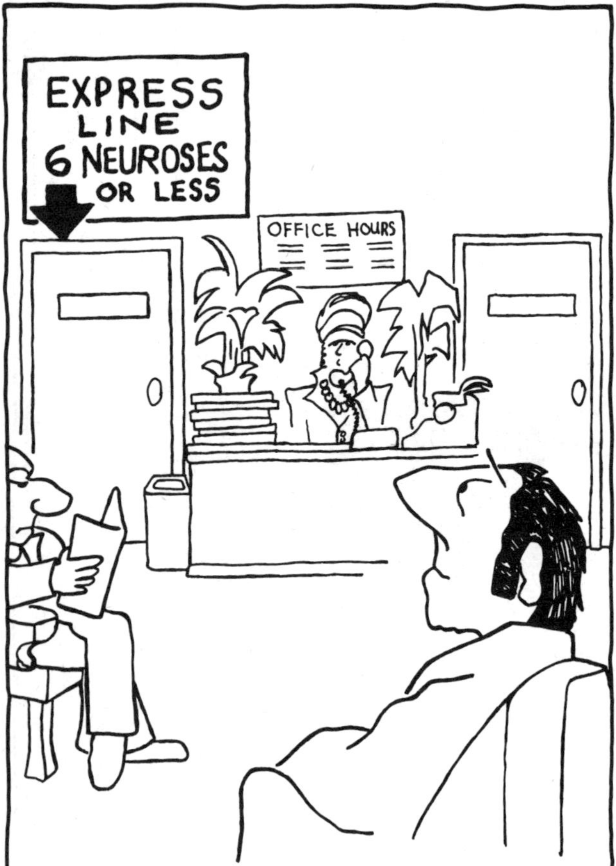
EXPRESS
LINE
6 NEUROSES
OR LESS
OFFICE HOURS

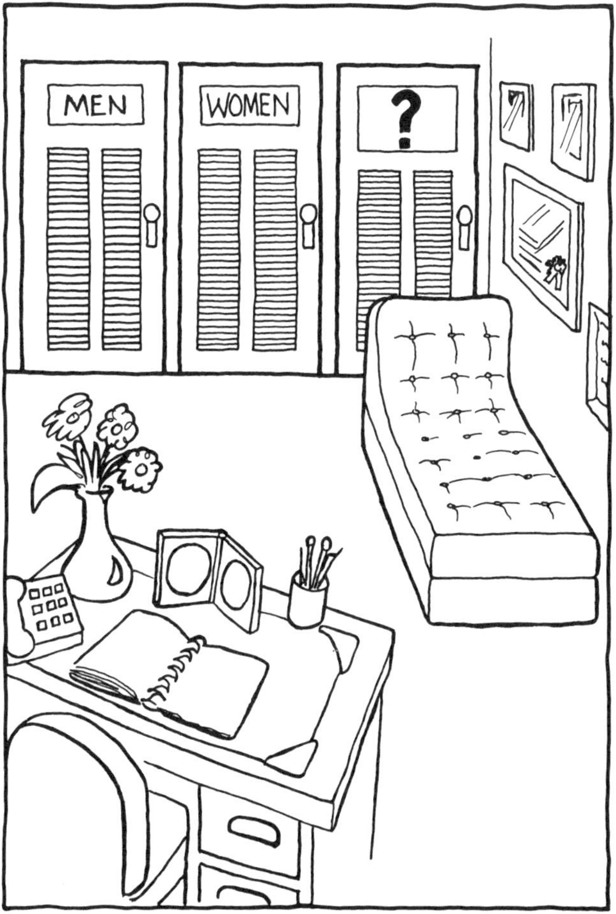
MEN
WOMEN
?

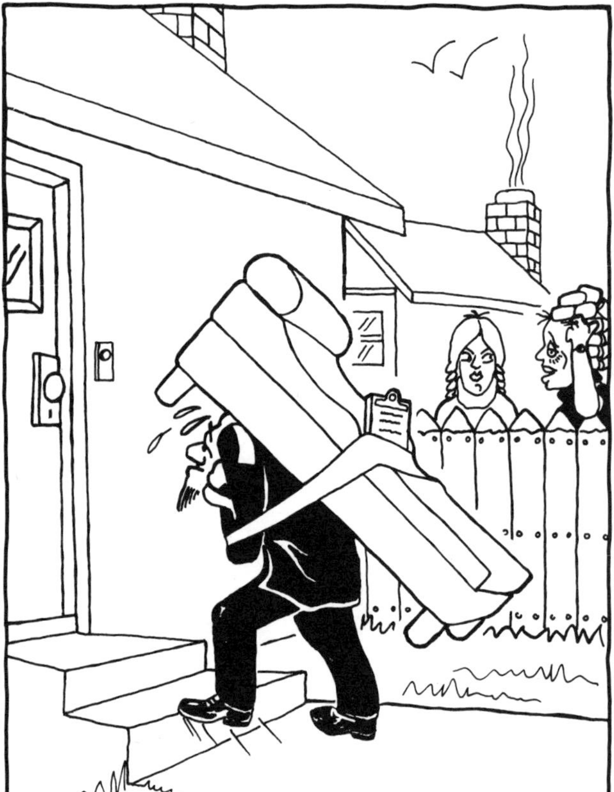

"I didn't know they made house calls."

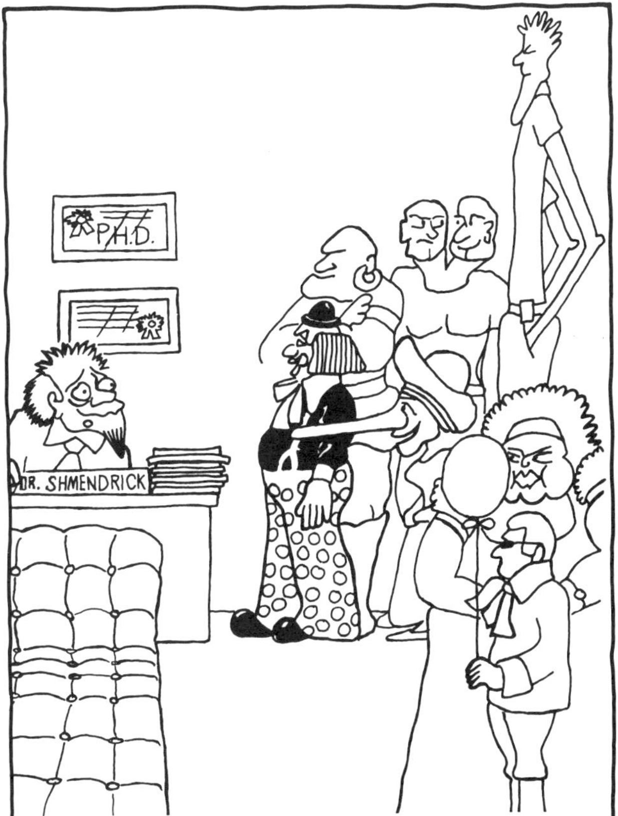

"We told our boss all about you....
of course you'll have to audition."

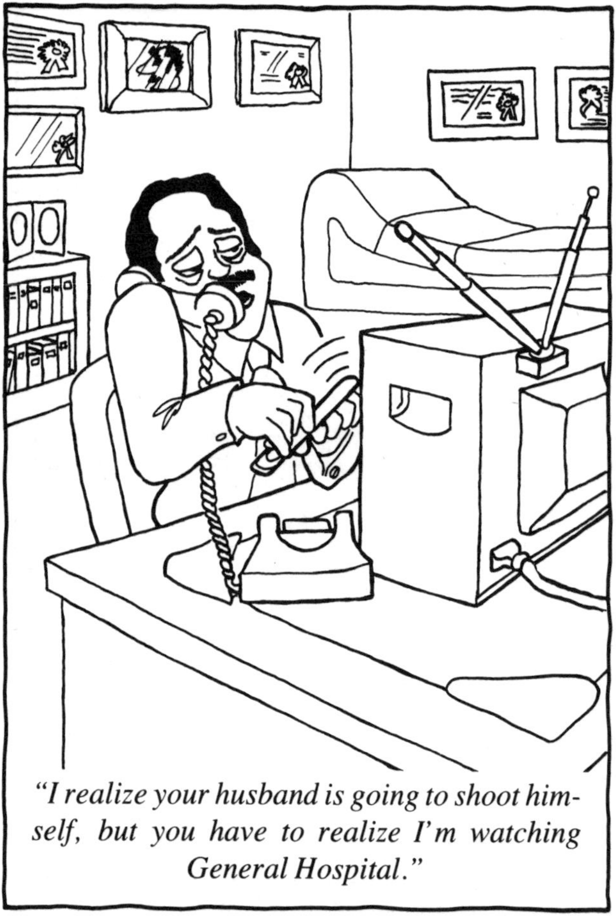

"I realize your husband is going to shoot himself, but you have to realize I'm watching General Hospital."

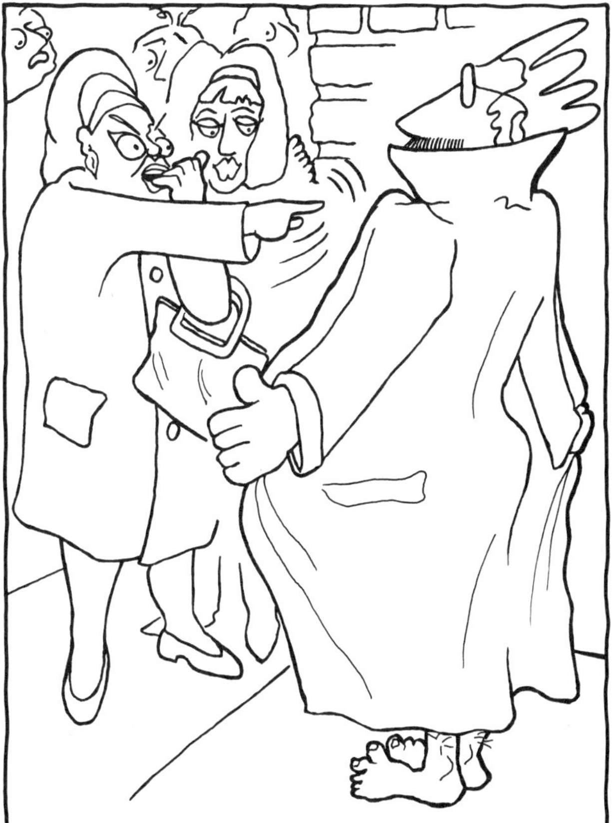

"Oh my God, that's my shrink!"

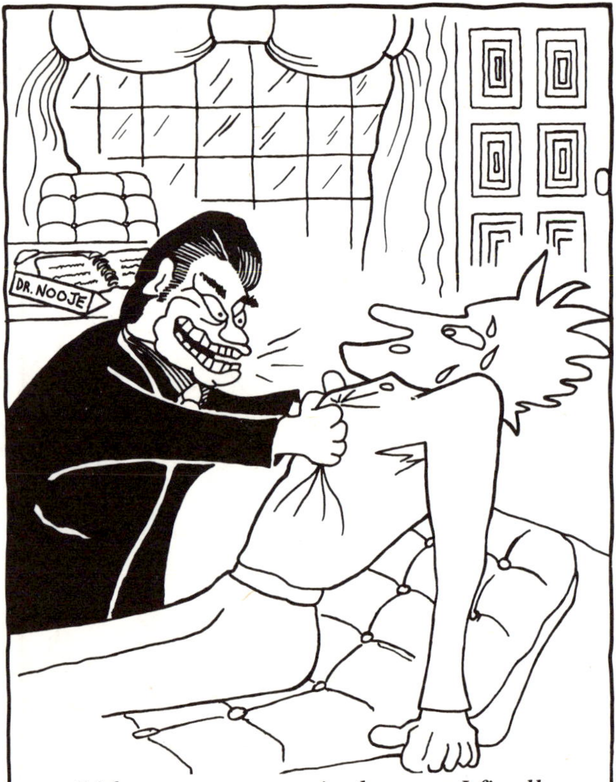

"After twenty years in therapy, I finally make you independent, and now you want to leave me?"